YOUR KNOWLEDGE HAS VALUE

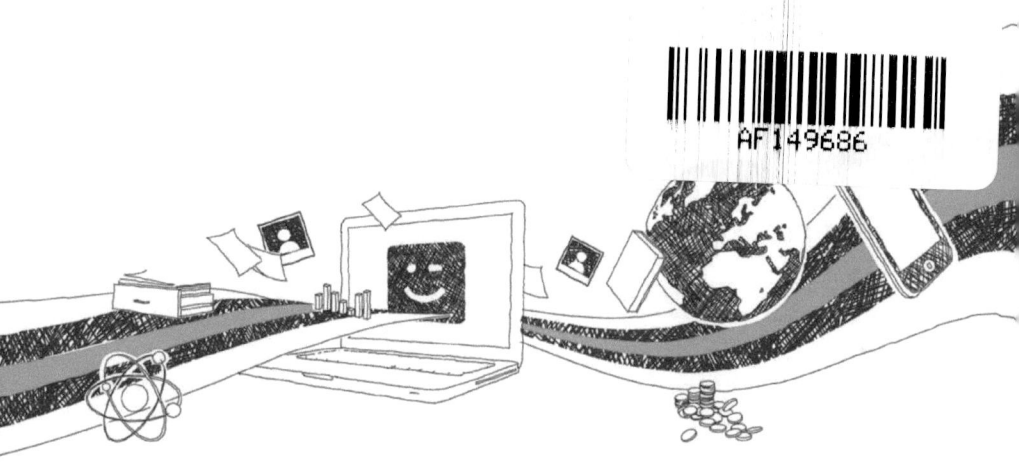

- We will publish your bachelor's and master's thesis, essays and papers

- Your own eBook and book - sold worldwide in all relevant shops

- Earn money with each sale

Upload your text at www.GRIN.com
and publish for free

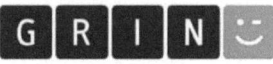

Pramesh Chalise

Comparative Study of Cryptosporidium Infestation in Wild Water Buffaloes (Bubalus arnee) and Domestic Buffaloes (Bubalus bubalis) of Koshi Tappu Wildlife Reserve

GRIN Verlag

Bibliografische Information der Deutschen Nationalbibliothek:

Die Deutsche Bibliothek verzeichnet diese Publikation in der Deutschen National-
bibliografie; detaillierte bibliografische Daten sind im Internet über http://dnb.d-
nb.de/ abrufbar.

Imprint:

Copyright © 2013 GRIN Verlag GmbH
Druck und Bindung: Books on Demand GmbH, Norderstedt Germany
ISBN: 978-3-656-62142-3

This book at GRIN:

http://www.grin.com/en/e-book/271150/comparative-study-of-cryptosporidium-
infestation-in-wild-water-buffaloes

1. Introduction

1.1 Background

Cryptosporidium species are coccidian, oocysts forming apicomplexan protozoa. They complete their life cycle both in humans and animals, through zoonotic and anthroponotic transmission resulting in disease state called as Cryptosporidiosis. They are frequent agents of gastrointestinal infection in humans, domestic animals, and other vertebrates. Three species of *Cryptosporidium* have been associated with infection in cattle. Two small-type oocysts, *C. parvum* and *C. bovis* (Fayer *et al.*, 2005), infect the small intestine. However, the larger type, *Cryptosporidium andersoni* that infects the abomasum has been implicated as a cause of reduced milk production in dairy cattle (Lindsay *et al.*, 2000).

Cryptosporidium parvum is the most frequently detected pathogen in calves less than 3 weeks age (Moore and Zeman, 1991; Fuente *et al.*, 1999), where it considered being one of the main common causes of diarrhea at this age (Koudela and Bokova 1997).

However, Cryptosporidiosis should not only be considered from the perspective of animal health and production; its zoonotic character and the possibility that animals may act as a source of infection to humans, via foodstuff and water, should also be considered. Although the infection leads to few deaths, serious economic losses can occur due to costs involved in the treatment (Graaf *et al.*, 1999). Single infection with *C. parvum* is usually present in diarrheic calves; however, mixed infection with other pathogens exaggerates the problem (Vanopdenbosch *et al.*, 1979).

Cryptosporidiosis in water buffaloes (*Bubalus bubalis*) received great interest in different localities of the world (Galiero *et al.*, 1994; Dubey *et al.*, 1992). The prevalence of Cryptosporidiosis was also mentioned in African buffaloes (*Syncerus caffer*) among wildlife animals in Tanzania (Mtambo *et al.*, 1997). However, the risk factors concerned with Cryptosporidiosis in buffalo calves have not been described.

1

The *Cryptosporidium spp.* infection has been recorded in over 170 animal species in 50 countries (Snelling *et al.*, 2007) in wide range of vertebrate hosts and humans, particularly in children (younger than 5 years old) and immunocompromised persons (Xiao *et al.*, 2004). *Cryptosporidium spp* are transmitted via faeco-oral route. The oocyst is the infective stage that is exceptionally resistant to environment stress and harsh chemical treatments, which allows the parasites to stably persist outside a host (Fayer *et al.*, 1997).

1.1.1 Classification

Phylum: Apicomplexa

Class: Sporozoasida

Subclass: Coccidiasina

Order: Eucooccidiida

Suborder: Eimeriina

Family: Cryptospordiidae (Ramirez *et al.*, 2004)

1.1.2 Pathogenesis

Little is known about the pathogenesis of the parasites and no safe and effective treatment has been successfully developed to combat Cryptosporidiosis. According to (Ramirez *et al.*, 2004), the life cycle of most *Cryptosporidium spp* completed within the gastrointestinal tract (primarily small intestine and colon) of the host, with developmental stages being associated with the luminal surface of the mucosal epithelial cells. Thick-wall oocysts are excreted from the infected host in fecal material and represent the infective stage of the parasite. Infection of *Cryptosporidium* in a new host results from the ingestion of these oocysts, which release sporozoites that invade the epithelial cells and undergo asexual and sexual multiplication to produce thin-walled and thick-walled oocysts. Thin-walled oocysts can excyst endogenously, resulting in autoinfection, which helps to explain the mechanism ofpersistent infections (in AIDS patients) in the absence of successive (thick-walled) oocysts exposure.

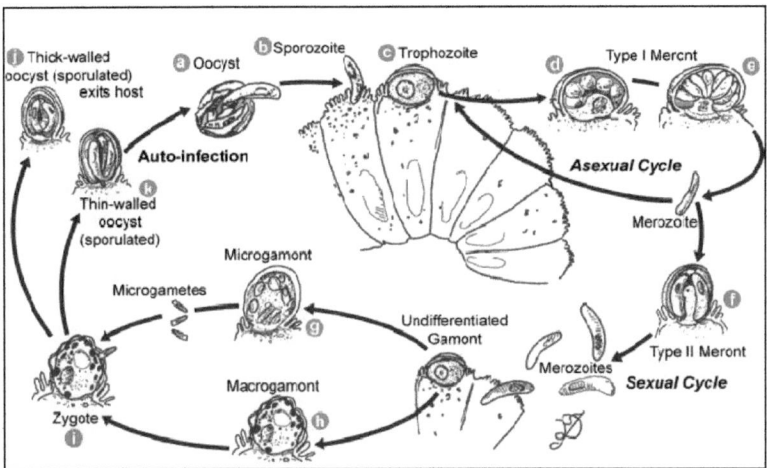

Figure – 1: Pathogenesis of *Cryptosporidium*.

Source: (Putignani and Menichella, 2010)

1.1.3Epidemiology

Unlike other intestinal pathogens, *Cryptosporidium* can infect several different hosts; can survive in most environments for long period of time due to its hardy cysts (Ramirez *et al*., 2004). It is an inhabitant of all climates and locales. In majority of cases the Cryptosporidiosis is diagnosed due to the presence of the oocysts and antigen in the faeces. Transmission of *Cryptosporidium* mainly occurs by ingestion of contaminated water (e.g. surface, drinking or recreational water), food sources (e.g. chicken salad, fruits, and vegetables) or by person-to-person contact (community and hospital infections). Zoonotic transmission of *C. parvum* occurs through exposure to infected animals (person-to-animal contact) or exposure to water (reservoir) contaminated by feces of infected animals (Putignani and Menchella, 2010).

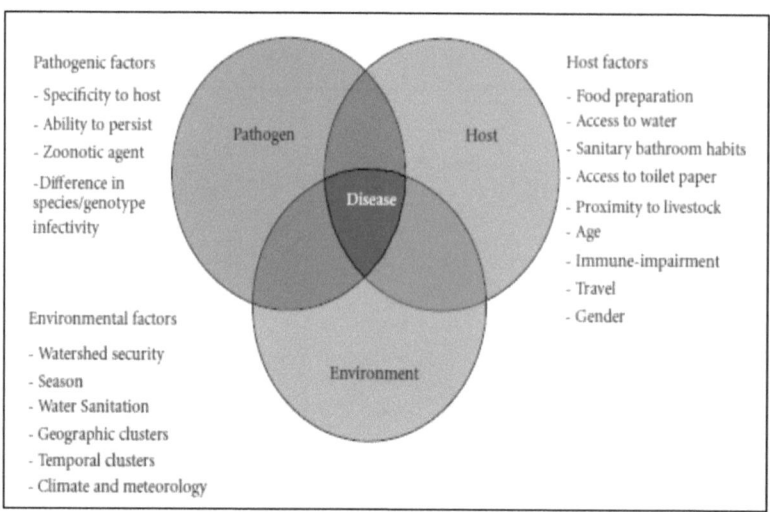

Pathogenic factors

- Specificity to host
- Ability to persist
- Zoonotic agent
- Difference in species/genotype infectivity

Environmental factors

- Watershed security
- Season
- Water Sanitation
- Geographic clusters
- Temporal clusters
- Climate and meteorology

Host factors

- Food preparation
- Access to water
- Sanitary bathroom habits
- Access to toilet paper
- Proximity to livestock
- Age
- Immune-impairment
- Travel
- Gender

Figure – 2: Epidemiology of *Cryptosporidium*

Source: (Putignani and Menichella, 2010)

Over 20 methods of staining aiming at the oocysts identification is applied in the microscopic diagnosis. However the microscopic methods frequently fail in the diagnosis of asymptomatic infection requiring the need of molecular techniques.

1.1.4 Transmission pattern

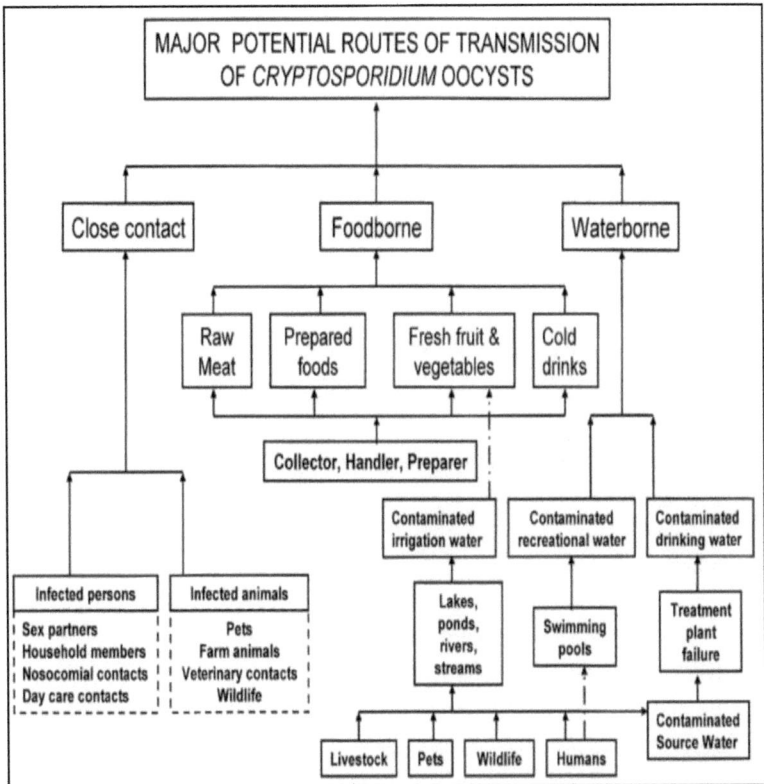

Figure – 3: Transmission pattern of *Cryptosporidium spp.*

1.2 Justification of the study

There is no single study regarding prevalence of cryptosporidiosis in wild water buffalo in Nepal, this study endeavors to bridge the knowledge gap in concerned field. Since the population of wild water buffalo is small and vulnerable, this kind of study helps towards the conservation efforts.

It is a guideline in our wild and domesticated buffalo population as it indicates the protozoan parasites infestation. Though the exact mortality of younger calves,

5

primarily the suckling ones is yet to be known. Cryptosporidiosis may be one of the killer diseases in young ones in our context.

1.3 Objectives of the study

1.3.1 General objective

- To study comparative prevalence of *Cryptosporidium species* in wild water and domestic buffaloes in Koshi Tappu wildlife reserve, Nepal.

1.3.2 Specific objectives

- To know the prevalence of *Cryptosporidium* in wild water and domestic buffaloes in Koshi Tappu Wildlife reserve, Nepal

- To make comparative analysis of the occurrence of *Cryptosporidium* in different seasons.

1.4Limitations of the study

- The study is just a cross sectional study. So the results can only be related to a point of time and this cannot be related to a period of time.
- Sample size and the species are limited due to which the results cannot be generalized for the entire population of the species in that area.
- The individual difference of the animals like immunity and resistance, among the animals may have some effects on the study.
- Genotyping for the species identification could not be done from the positive samples.

2. Literature review

Venu *et al.*, 2012 investigates prevalence of *Cryptosporidium* through molecular methods and found 39.65% prevalence in the southern states of India with predisposition in females than males and in young age.

Siwila and Mwape, 2012 used similar methods as this research and found out the total prevalence to be 44.4 % with the presence of parasite in every farms investigated.

Jeníkova *et al.*, 2011 identified two species, *C. suis* and *C. pig* genotype II as major causative agent of the cryptosporidiosis in piglets. It was further indicated that the *C. suis* was found in all 1-12 week age piglets whereas, *Cryptosporidium pig* genotype II was recorded only in animals older than 6 week of age.

Chen *et al.*, 2011 identified *Cryptosporidium* in all 12 pig farms under study and varying in the prevalence from 14.1 to 90.6%.

Ghimire *et al.*, 2010 reported a case of *Cryptosporidium* infection from environmental contamination in swimming pools in Nepal.

Among animals, the wild animal had the highest prevalence and was observed in deer which was 71% and followed by rhino 25%. The calves and buffalo calves were suffering from 34 and 37% respectively (Karna, 2010).

Khan *et al.*, 2010 identifies age related pattern of the *Cryptosporidium* infection and also the *C.hominis*, *C. parvum* and *C. bovis* were identified from farm workers in India which clarifies a potential risk of zoonotic transmission between cattle and humans on dairy farms.

Amatya *et al.*, 2010 identified 4.4% prevalence in the HIV seronegative children from eastern region of Nepal. Ghimire, Mishra and Sherchand, 2005 identified

Cryptosporidium in 11.3% of 9000 stool samples. They found out 16.7% positive in washings of radishes, 3.3% in cauliflower, and 13.3% in washings of mustard leaves washed in the rivers of Kathmandu. Furthermore, 13.0% in sewage water, 9.0% in river water and 0% in pond water and 1% in well water was demonstrated. Dhakal*et al.*, 2004 identified *C. parvum* in 10.4 % children from Kanti children hospital.

Mallinath *et al.*, 2009 investigated the cryptosporidiosis in adult bovines in organized dairy farms and Paul *et al.*, 2009 investigated 12.85% prevalence in over all parts of India, with highest occurrence in the northern states of the country. This shows that Nepal being attached to the northern part of India, posses risk of the *Cryptosporidium* infection.

Studies done by Mandal and Singh, 2009, reported the prevalence of the *Cryptosporidium* in cow calves, buffalo calves, adult cows and adult buffaloes of IAAS livestock farm as 60%, 70%, 30% and 30% respectively.

Yatswako *et al.*, 2007 investigated *Cryptosporidium*oocysts from the pig in Nigeria and reported 13.9% positive with 18.7% of the associated human population to be positive suggesting the potential zoonotic transmission. Another work by Fayer *et al.*, 2007 observed a very low prevalence of this parasite in adult cattle as compared to young ones.

The American Bison (*Bison bison*) sometimes occupies grazing lands on or adjacent to those occupied by beef cattle, and some bison are raised for meat in the United States and Canada. *Cryptosporidium* has been detected in both the American and European bison (*B. bonasus*) at the Lisbon and Barcelona Zoos (Gómez *et al.*, 2000; Alves *et al.*, 2005). Surprisingly, the isolate from the American Bison at the Lisbon Zoo was *Cryptosporidium* mouse genotype (Alves *et al.*, 2005). Out of 31 outbreak cases (2004), 16 were from School outbreaks, 8 from school trip outbreaks and 3 from religious ceremony outbreaks (Ghimire *et al.*, 2005).

Cryptosporidium was reported that very high prevalence of *C. parvum* was found in the different parts of Nepal such as Jomsom (17%), Kathmandu valley (17.5%) and Chitwan (14.6%). It was more commonly seen during warm rainy season, which

8

reflects the increased oocysts contamination of surface and domestic water supplies in this period (Ghimire *et al.*, 2005).

Santin *et al.*, 2004 investigated *Cryptosporidium* in 971 calves and found 35.5% positive and higher proportion to be present in pre weaned than post weaned calves. *Cryptosporidium* was identified in from all the farms. Water buffalo (*Bubalus sp.*) are economically important animals raised for draft, meat, and milk in many parts of the world.

Ramirez *et al.*, 2004 stated in a review paper that comparative studies between bovine and human Cryptosporidiosis revealed that zoonotic transmission of the disease is going on.

Ghimire *et al.*, 2004 examined 148 stool specimens collected from 75 confirmed cases of HIV/AIDS to assess the prevalence of cryptosporidiosis in patients with HIV and AIDS. The specimens were analyzed using Kinyoun-modified acid fast staining. Cryptosporidiosis was found in 10.7% of the total 75 cases studied. Out of 75 cases, 30.7% (23) suffered from diarrhea, of which *Cryptosporidium parvum* accounted for 34.8% (8) cases. Matos *et al.*, 1998 reported the findings of a longitudinal observational study on HIV infected patients in Santa Maria Hospital, Lisbon grouped by presumed transmission group, who had diarrhea. Modified formyl-ether concentration followed by modified Ziehl-Neelsen and phenol-auramine/carbol-fuchsin staining techniques were used to identify *Cryptosporidium* from 465 patients. Cryptosporidiosis was reported in 36/465 (8% and 95%: Confidence Interval 6-10) patients. Gupta, Sinha and Raizada, 2008 found the infection in 25% of the HIV infected patients in Gujarat. Similarly Taherkhani *et al.*, 2007 demonstrated 26.7% infection rate in the AIDS patients of Iran.

Sherchand and Shrestha, 1996 screened three hundred and fifty-four soft, loose or watery stool specimens from patients in Nepal with acute diarrhea were for the presence of *Cryptosporidium* oocysts. A modified Ziehl Neelsen with DMSO staining method was used for detecting *Cryptosporidium* oocysts in the stool samples. The oocysts were identified in 24 (6.8%) samples, while 46 samples (13%) showed mixed infections.

9

Treatment of Cryptosporidiosis is not effective in cattle. So, control measures are mainly based on preventive measures rather than treatment (Woods *et al.*, 1996). However, halofuginone lactate was found to have anti-cryptosporidial effect (Jarvie *et al.*, 2005; Klein, 2007). Furthermore, *Cryptosporidium* oocysts are resistant to the commonly used disinfectant at recommended concentrations (Campbell *et al.*, 1982). It is necessary to find management approaches to minimize the risk of infection with cryptosporidiosis.

Cryptosporidium oocysts were detected in feces of water buffalo in Italy, Brazil, Cuba, Egypt, and India (Canestri-Trotti and Quesada, 1983; Canestri-Trotti *et al.*, 1984; Galiero *et al.*, 1994; Iskander *et al.*, 1987; Rodríguez Diego *et al.*, 1991; Dubey *et al.*, 1992; Araujo *et al.*, 1996). The prevalence of infection ranged from 6 to 39%.

Garcia *et al.*, 1993 and Kaminijolo *et al.*, 1993 recorded 27.8% and 19.6% *Cryptosporidium* in cattle. Gracia*et al.*, 1993 found 31.4% and 21.62% on diarrheic and non diarrheic cases positive for *Cryptosporidium* oocyst in Brazil.

One study found a higher incidence of infection in diarrheic buffalo; another found no conclusive relationship (Dubey *et al.*, 1992; Galiero *et al.*, 1994). Of 616 and 525 buffalo examined in Cuba and Egypt, respectively, oocysts were found only in calves (Abou-Eisha, 1994; Rodríguez Diego *et al.*, 1991).

Dubey *et al.*, 1990 reviewed the incidence of cryptosporidiosis in the diarrheic bovine cases from different parts of the world. They recorded 45.5% incidence in USA, 24.5% in U.K. 26% in U.S.S.R. 40% in Germany and 27% in Hungary.

3. Materials and methods

3.1 Study area

The study was conducted in KoshiTappu wildlife Reserve, Nepal.

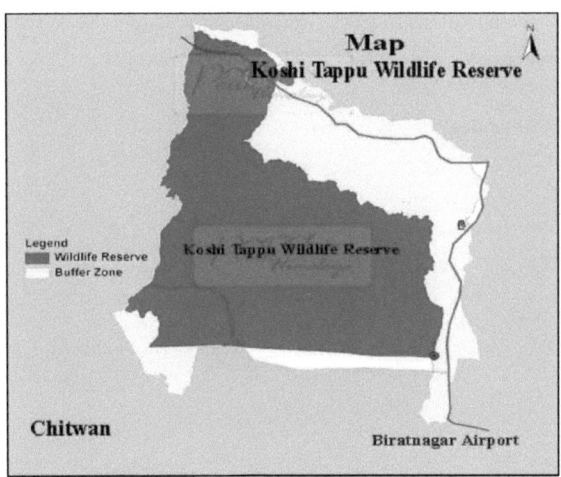

Figure - 4: Map of study area

3.2 Methods of sampling

Random sampling technique was used to collect dung sample.

3.3 Sample Size

Dung samples from 100 wild water buffaloes and 100 domestic buffaloes living near the periphery of river basins of Sapta Koshi were examined for the presence of *Cryptosporidium*. For pre-monsoon and post-monsoon study, equal number of samples, i.e 50 samples each was collected respectively.

3.4 Sample collection

The dung samples were collected from the farms in the river basins of Sapta Koshi, concentrating on Buffer Zone of KTWR. Rectal collection was carried out early morning in domestic buffalo using the sterilized gloves whereas random purposive collection of the wild water buffalo was made. The samples were collected in the zip-lock plastic sample bags and labeled accordingly which included sample identification and site of collection. The collected samples were transported in the ice cooled box in order to maintain low temperature of the samples. The transported samples were kept in the refrigeration in the parasitology lab AHRD of NARC until processing.

3.5 Sample Processing/Methodology

3.5.1 Materials

- Plastic ball pipette
- Centrifuge
- Centrifuge tube
- Tea strainer
- Dung sample
- Electronic balance
- Slides
- Distilled water
- Laboratory Sodium Chloride (393 g/L)
- Methanol
- Carbol fuchsin
- Acid alcohol (3%)
- Malachite green (5%)
- Oil emersion microscope
- Oil

The samples were stained by Ziehl-Nelson Staining technique after Modified Sheather concentration technique using centrifugation (Zhang *et al.*, 2012; Zajac and Conboy, 2006).

3.5.2 Preparation of smear

- 5 g of the collected dung sample was put in 10 ml of the distilled water and mixed well.
- 20 ml of the supersaturated solution of Nacl (393 g/L) was added to the solution.
- This mixture was centrifuged at 2000 rpm for 15 minutes and the supernatant was taken.
- Distilled water was added to the supernatant and the final volume was made up to 100 ml adding the distilled water.
- This solution was now centrifuged at 5000 rpm for 15 minutes.
- The supernatant was discarded and the sediment was taken using glass rod and smear on the glass slide was prepared which is air dried.
- The air dried glass slide was fixed with methanol and set for staining.

3.5.3 Staining of smear slide by modified Ziehl Neelsen stain method

- The air dried smear was fixed with methanol for 5 minutes.
- Then smear was stained with unheated Carbol fuchsin for 7 minutes and washed off with distilled water.
- After that decolorized with 3% acid alcohol for 10-15 seconds (one dip) and washed off with water.
- Than the slide was counter stained with 0.5% malachite green for 30 seconds and again washed off with water.
- Finally the smear was examined microscopically for oocysts, using a low power magnification to detect the oocysts and the oil immersion objective to identify them.

3.5.4 Data analysis

The obtained data were tabulated and analyzed by using statistical tool (Chi square) and Microsoft Excel.

4. Results

4.1 Overall prevalence

Of the 100 dung samples collected from wild water buffaloes and domestic buffaloes respectively, were analyzed microscopically by acid-fast stained. All the coprological laboratory works were conducted at AHRD, NARC. Out of 200 samples, 6% were positive for the oocysts of cryptosporidium.

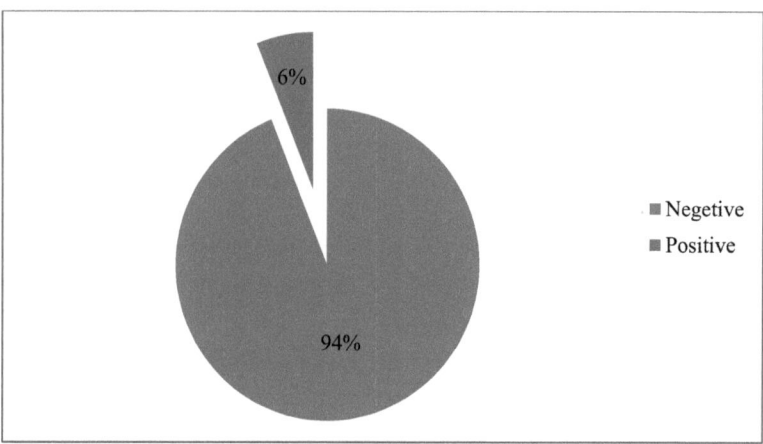

Figure – 5: Overall prevalence of *Cryptosporidium*

Table – 1: Chi square test between species and season

Variables	Labels	Positive	Negative	Total	P value
Species	Wild buffalo	7	93	100	χ2= 0.3546
	Domestic buffalo	5	95	100	P=0.551515
Season	Pre-monsoon	1	99	100	χ2= 8.8652
	Post-monsoon	11	89	100	P=0.002907*

* Statistically significant difference at 5% level of significance.

14

4.2 Season wise prevalence

For a comparative study between two seasons pre-monsoon and post-monsoon period were taken in consideration. Pre-monsoon dung collection was taken in June while Post-Monsoon dung was collected in the month of October.

4.2.1 Pre-monsoon

50 dung samples from wild water buffalo and domestic buffalo were collected respectively. Out of 100 samples, 1 (1%) was positive for the oocysts of *Cryptosporidium*.

4.2.2 Post-monsoon

50 dung samples from wild water buffalo and domestic buffalo were collected respectively. Out of 100 samples, 11 (11%) were positive for the oocysts of *Cryptosporidium*.

Seasons had a significant effect ($p < 0.05$, $\chi 2 = 8.8652$) on the prevalence of infection with the higher prevalence in post-monsoon (11 %) as compared to pre-monsoon.

Table –2: Season wise prevalence

Season	Sample Size	Total Positive
Pre-monsoon	100	1
Post-monsoon	100	11
Total	200	12

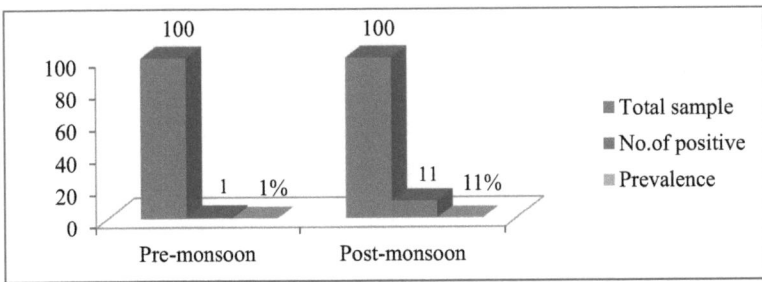

Figure – 6: Season wise prevalence

15

4.3 Species wise prevalence

Among 100 dung samples from wild water buffalo and domestic buffalo, microscopy results shows 7% and 5% positive respectively.Statistically insignificant higher prevalence of *Cryptosporidium spp.* was recorded in wild water buffalo than domestic buffalo (p < 0.05, $\chi 2$=0.3546).

Table – 3: Species wise prevalence

Species	Sample Size	Total Positive
Wild Buffalo	100	7
Domestic Buffalo	100	5
Total	200	12

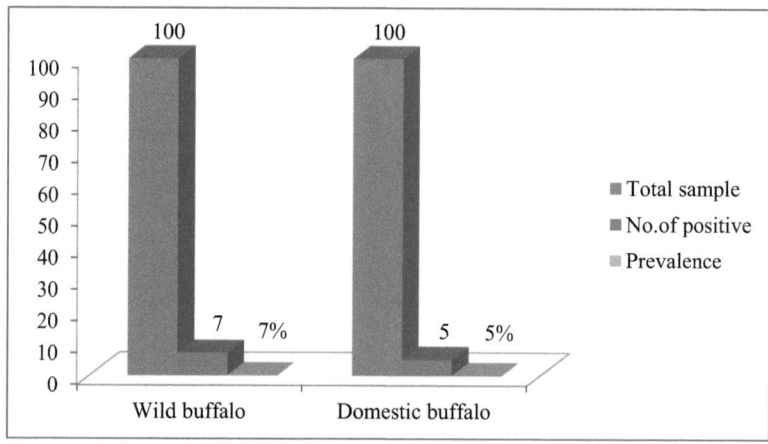

Figure – 7: Species wise prevalence

Table – 4: Species and Season wise prevalence

Species	Pre Monsoon			Post Monsoon		
	Sample Size	Positive	Negative	Sample Size	Positive	Negative
Wild Buffalo	50	1	49	50	6	44
Domestic buffalo	50	0	50	50	5	45
Total	100	1	99	100	11	89

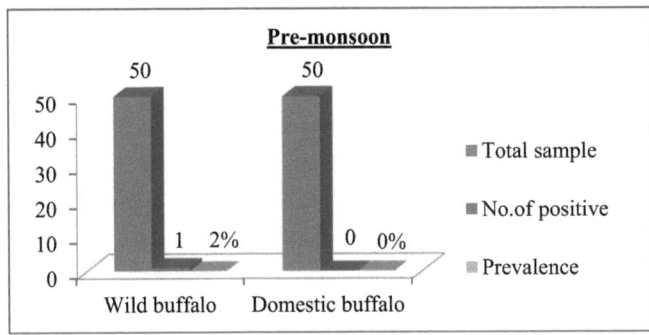

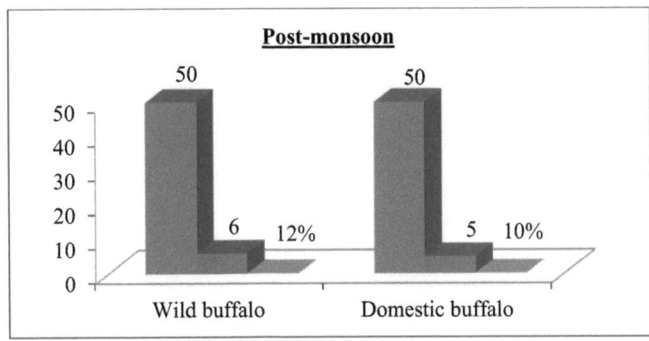

Figure – 8: Species and Season wise prevalence

17

5. Discussion

The objective of the present study was to describe the prevalence and comparative study associated with cryptosporidiosis in wild water buffalo in KTWR-BZ and its vulnerability due to close association with domestic buffalo in terms of sharing same habitat. Single remnant population of wild water buffalo is confined only in KTWR. Since there is no single study regarding prevalence of cryptosporidiosis in wild water buffalo in Nepal, this study endeavors to bridge the knowledge gap in concerned field. Since the population of wild water buffalo is small and vulnerable, this kind of study helps towards the conservation efforts.

Cattle worldwide are infected with *Cryptosporidium* causing morbidity and mortality resulting primarily in diarrhea, and resulting in the most severe infections in immune-compromised individuals. The highest prevalence has been identified in pre-weaned calves (Condoleo *et al.*, 2007). However, difficulties during collection of samples from wild buffaloes did not facilitate the sample according to age and sex which were not considered in this study. A close association between livestock and feral rodents facilitates transmission of *C. parvum* between these hosts and ensures its perpetuation. So, a similar study is essential to understand a pattern of prevalence of *cryptosporidium* between domestic buffalo and wild water buffalo.

Paul *et al.*, 2009 investigated 12.85% prevalence in over all parts of India, with highest occurrence in the northern states of the country. This shows that Nepal being neighbor to the northern part of India, possess risk of the *Cryptosporidium* infection in its wild as well as domestic population.

According to this study, the overall prevalence of *cryptosporidium* was 6% while *cryptosporidium* infection in wild water buffalo and domestic buffalo is 7% and 5% respectively. The present study also shows similar pattern of prevalence as study carried out in wild water buffalo in India and Italy by (Dubey *et al.*, 1992 and Galiero *et al.*, 1994) respectively have the prevalence ranged from 6% to 39%.However, in domestic buffalo our study shows a lower prevalence than study of (Venu *et al.*, 2012) in southern state of India which shows 39.65% and study of (Paul *et al.*, 2009) of overall India shows 12.85%. The lower prevalence of *cryptosporidium* in our study may be due to the small sample size which is a result of small population size of wild water buffalo counting 237 in KTWR (DNPWC, 2011). Similarly reared population of domestic buffalo was low in the study area and frequently the buffaloes were sold.

In the study, more animals were infected in post-monsoon (6% wild water buffalo and 5% domestic buffalo) than in pre-monsoon. Seasons had a significant effect (p < 0.05) on the prevalence of infection with the higher prevalence in post-monsoon (11%) as compared to pre-monsoon. (Mayura *et al.*, 2013) also support that season play an important role in infection. The reason for higher incidence in post-monsoon may be that *Cryptosporidium* multiply faster in hot and humid condition and their life cycle accelerate in wet environment.

There are no previous reports on the presence of this infection in wild water buffalo and domestic buffalo in Nepal. In the present study, the prevalence of *Cryptosporidium* spp. infection in Wild water buffalo and domestic buffalo were 7% and 5% respectively. The present investigation seems to be the first report on the presence of this infection in both wild water buffalo and domestic buffalo from Nepal. Statistically insignificant higher prevalence of *Cryptosporidium spp.* was recorded in wild water buffalo than domestic buffalo (p < 0.05). This may be due to equal susceptibility and tolerance in both.

The grazing pasture land for both the species are nearly same during dry and winter months. Animals may have picked up the infection during that time hence for the prevalence of the protozoan parasite is nearly equal and is not significant.

The importance of the comparative study of *cryptosporidium* infestation in wild water buffalo and domestic buffalo of Koshi Tappu wildlife reserve is a guideline in our wild and domestic buffalo population as it indicates the protozoan parasites infestation. Though the exact mortality of younger calves, primarily the suckling ones is yet to be known, cryptosporidiosis may be one of the killer diseases in young ones in our context. Further works and study should be carried out in this regard with more sample size considering all the seasons.

6. Conclusion and Recommendation

6.1 Conclusion

This is one of the first research which may establishes river as an epidemiological factor for the transmission of *Cryptosporidium spp.* in Nepal. Wild buffalo and domestic buffalo lie in the same epidemiological cycle of the protozoan parasites. Furthermore, this research reports *Cryptosporidium* in wild buffalo and domesticbuffalo for the first time in Nepal.

Cryptosporidium was found to be prevalent in the wild buffalo and domestic buffalo in the periphery of the SaptaKoshi river basins. Higher prevalence rate was observed in wild buffalo than in domestic buffalo in this research. Seasonality variation was also studied in which prevalence of *cryptosporidium* in post-monsoon was significant to that of pre-monsoon samples collected. Further study should be carried out in this regard with more sample size considering all season. For the accurate results regarding the prevalence and situation on the whole population, research involving adequate sample size and using molecular techniques should be carried out.

6.2 Recommendation

- Frequent research should be carried out in wild animals in different national parks and wildlife reserves.
- Wildlife expertise along with veterinary doctor should be appointed in national parks and wildlife reserves.
- Direct contact between wild water buffalo and domestic buffalo should be minimized through solar fencing on national park boundaries to minimize risk of disease transmission.

References

Abou-Eisha, A. M. 1994. Cryptosporidial infection in man and faro animals in Ismailia Governorate.*Vet. Med. J. Giza,* **42**: 107–111.

Alves, M., Xiao, L., Lemos, V., Zhou, L., Cama, V., Cunha, M. B., Matos, O., and Antunes, F. 2005. Occurrence and molecular characterization of *Cryptosporidium* in mammals and reptiles at the Lisbon Zoo. *Parasitol. Re,* **97**: 108–112.

Amatya, R., Poudyal, N., Gurung, R., Khanal. B., 2010. Prevalence of *Cryptosporidium species* in paediatric patients in Eastern Nepal. Tropical Doctor.

Araujo, M. D., Paiva, G. S., Antunes, R. L., Chaplin E. E. and Silva, N. R. S. 1996. Occurrence of *Cryptosporidium parvum* and *Cryptosporidium muris* in buffalos *(Bubalus bubalis)* at Amapa state, Brazil. *Arq. Fac. Vet. UFRG,* **24**: 85–90.

Campbell, I., Tzipori, A. S., Hutchison, G., and Angus, K. W. 1982. Effect of disinfectants on survival of *Cryptosporidium* oocysts. Veterinary Record, **111**: 414–415.

Canestri-Trotti, G. and Quesada, A. 1983. First report of *Cryptosporidium* in Italian water buffalos. *Estratto da Attidella Società Italiana delle Scienze Veterinarie,* **37**: 737–740.

Canestri-Trotti, G., Quesada, A. and Visconti, S. 1984. Ricerchesulla fauna protozoa riai ntestinale del buffalo (*Bubalus bubalis*). *Estrattodagli Attidella Società Italiana di Buiatria*, **16**: 433–450.

Chen, Z., R. Mi, H. Yu, Y. Shi, Y. Huang, Y. Chen, P. Zhou, Y. Cai and J. Lin. 2011. Prevalence of *Cryptosporidiumspp*. In pigs in Shanghai, China.*Veterinary Parasitology*, **181**: 113-119.

Condoleo, R. U., Rinaldi, L., Saralli, G., Morgoglione, M. E.,Schioppi, M., Condoleo, R., Musella, V., Cringoli G. 2007. An updating on *Cryptosporidium parvum* in the water buffalo. *Ital. J. Anim. Sci.*, **6** (2): 917-919.

Dhakal, D. N., Rajendra, B. C., Sherchand, J. B., and Mishra, P. N. 2004. *Cryptosporidium parvum*: An observational study in Kanti Children Hospital, Kathamandu, Nepal. *Journal of Nepal Health Research Council*, **2** (1):1-5

DNPWC. 2011. Arna (Asian wild buffalo) census Report 2068 (Ashok Ram), pp 20.

Dubey, J. P., Fayer, R. and Rao, J. R. 1992. Crytosporidialoocysts in faeces of water buffalo and zebu calves in India. *J. Vet*, **6**: 55–56.

Dubey, J. P., Frayer, R., and Speer, C. R. 1990. Cryptosporidiosis in man and animals. CRC Press, Boca Raton, Florida. pp: 65-93.

Fayer, R., M., Santin and J. M., Trout. 2007. Prevalence of *Cryptosporidium Species* and genotypes in mature dairy cattle on farms in eastern United States compared with younger cattle from the same locations. *Veterinary Parasitology*, **145**: 260-266.

Fayer, R., Santin, M., Xiao, L., 2005. *Cryptosporidium bovis* and *spp* (*Apicomplexa: Cryptosporidiidae*) in cattle (*Bos Taurus*). *Journal of parasitology*, **91**: 624–629.

Fayer, R., Speer, C. A., Dubey, J. P., 1997. The general biology of *Cryptosporidium*, p. 1-41. In R. E. Fayer. *Cryptosporidium* and Cryptosporidiosis, CRC Press, inc., Boca Raton, Florida.

Fuente, R., Luzón, M., Ruiz-Santa-Quiteria, J. A., García, A., Cid, D., Orden, J. A., García, S., Sanz, R., Gómez- Bautista, M. 1999. *Cryptosporidium* and concurrent infections with other major enteropathogens in 1–30 day old diarrheic dairy calves in central Spain. *Veterinary Parasitology*, **80**: 179–185.

Galiero, G., Consalvo, F. and Carullo, M. 1994. Cryptosporidiosis in buffalo calves; *Sel.Vet*, **35**: 449–453.

Ghimire, P., Sapkota, D. and Manandhar,S. P. 2004. Cryptosporidiosis: opportunistic infection in HIV/AIDS patients in Nepal. *Journal of Tropical Medical Parasitology*, **27**: 7-10.

Ghimire, T. R., Ghimire, L. V.,Shahu, R. K. and Mishra, P. N 2010. *Cryptosporidium* and Cyclospora infection transmission by swimming. *Journal of Institute of Medicine,* **32** (1): 43-45.

Ghimire, T. R., Mishra, P. N. and Sherchand, J. B.2005. The seasonal outbreaks of Cyclospora and *Cryptosporidium* in Kathmandu, Nepal.*Journal of Nepal Health Research Council*, **3** (1): 39-48.

Gómez M. S., Torres, J., Gracenea, M., Fernández-Morán, J. and González-Moreno, O. 2000. Further report on *Cryptosporidium* in Barcelona zoo mammals. *Parasitol. Res*, **86**: 318–323.

Graaf, D. C., Vanopdenbosch, E., Ortega-Mora, L. M., Abbassi, H., Peeters, J. E. 1999. A review of the importance of cryptosporidiosis in farm animals. *International Journal of Parasitology*, **29**: 1269–1287.

Gracia, A. M. and Lima, J. D. 1993. Frequency of *Cryptosporidium* in suckling dairy calves. *Arquivo-Brasileiro-de-Medicina-Veterinaria-e-Zootecia,* **45** (2): 193-198.

Gupta, M., Sinha, M. and Raizada, N. 2008. Opportunistic intestinal protozoan parasitic infection in HIV positive patient in Jamnagar, Gujarat. SAARC *Journal of Tuberculosis Lung Diseases & HIV/AIDS*. **1**: 1-4

Iskander, A. R., TawfeeK, A., Farid, A. F. 1987. Cryptosporidial infection among buffalo calves in Egypt. *Indian Journal of Animal Science*, pp **57**, 1057.

Jarvie, B. D., Trotz-Williams, L. A., McKnight, D. R., Leslie, K. E., Wallace, M. M., Todd, C. G., Sharpe, P. H., Peregrine, A. S. 2005. Effect of halofuginone lactate on the occurrence of *Cryptosporidium parvum* and growth of neonatal dairy calves. *Journal of Dairy Science*, **88**: 1801–6.

Jenikova, M., K. Nemejc, B. Sak, D. Kvetonova and M. Kvac. 2011. New view on the age specificity of pig *Cryptosporidium* by species-specific primers for distinguishing *Cryptosporidium suis* and *Cryptosporidium* pig genotype II. *Veterinary Parasitology*, **176**: 120-125.

Kaminijolo, J.S., Adesiyun, A. A., Loregnard, R. and Kitson-Piggott, W. 1993. Prevelence of *Cryptosporidium* oocysts in livestock in Trinidad and Tobago.*Vet. Parasitol*, **45** (3-5): 209-213

Karna S.R. 2010. Prevalence of *Cryptosporidium* in domestic animals (calves of cattle and buffaloes), captive elephants, wild animals (Rhinoceros and Deer) and HIV/AIDS patients in some villages of buffer zone of Chitwan National Park. A B.V.Sc & A.H. Internship thesis submitted to Tribhuvan University.

Khan, S. M., Debnath, C., Pramanik, A. M., Xiao, L., Nozak, T. and Ganguly, S. 2010. Molecular characterization and assessment of zoonotic transmission of *Cryptosporidium* from dairy cattle in West Bengal, India. *Veterinary Parasitology*, **171**: 41-47.

Klein, P., 2007. Preventive and therapeutic efficacy of halofuginone- lactate against *Cryptosporidium parvum* in spontaneously infected calves: A centralised, randomised, double-blind, placebo-controlled study.

Koudela, B., Bokova, A., 1997. The effect of cotrimoxazole on experimental *Cryptosporidium parvum* infection in kids. *Veterinary Research*, **28**: 405–412.

Lindsay, D. S., Upton, S. J., Owens, D. S., Morgan, U. M., Mead, J. R., Blagburn, B. L., 2000. *Cryptosporidium andersoni (Apicomplexa: Cryptosporiidae) from cattle, Bostaurus.Journal of Eukaryotes Microbiology*, **47**: 91–95.

Mallinath, R. H. K., P. G. Chikkachowdappa, A. K. J. Gowda and P. E. D Souza. 2009. *Studies on the prevalence of cryptosporidiosis in bovines in organized dairy farms in and around Bangalore, South India.* Veterinary Archive, **79**: 461-470.

Mandal, B. N. and D. K. Singh. 2009. Internship Report. *Prevalence of Cryptosporidium spp. in cows and buffaloes of IAAS livestock Farm*, pp: 27

Matos, O., Tomás, A., Aguiar, P., Casemore, D. and Antunes, F. 1998. *Prevalence of cryptosporidiosis in aids patients with diarrhea insantamaria hospital, lisbon.*

Maurya, P. S., Rakesh, R., Pradeep, B., Kumar, S., Kundu, K., Garg, R., Ram, H., Kumar, A., Banerjee, P. S. 2013. Prevalence and risk factors associated with *Cryptosporidium spp.* infection in young domestic livestock in India. *Trop Anim Health Prod (2013)*, **45**: 941–946.

Moore, D. A., Zeman, D. H., 1991. Cryptosporidiosis in neonatal calves: 277 cases (1986–1987). *Journal of American Veterinary Medical Association*, **19**: 1969–1971.

Mtambo, M. M., Sebatwale, J. B., Kambarage, D. M., Muhairwa, A. P., Maeda, G. E., Kusiluka, L. J., Kazwala, R. R. 1997. *Prevalence of Cryptosporidium spp. oocysts in cattle and wildlife in Morogoro region, Tanzania.* Preventive Veterinary Medicine, **31**: 185–90.

Paul, S., Chandra, D., Tewari, A. K., Banerjee, P. S., Ray, D. D., Raina O. K. and Rao, J. R. 2009. Prevalence of *Cryptosporidium andersoni*: A molecular epidemiological survey among cattle in India.*Veterinary Parasitology*, **161**: 31-35.

25

Putignani, L. and Menichella, D. 2010. *Global Distribution, Public Health and Clinical Impact of the protozoan pathogen Cryptosporidium. International Perspectives on Infectious Diseases.* Article ID 753512, pp 39.

Ramirez, N. E., Ward, L. A. and Sreevatsan, S. 2004. *A review of the biology and epidemiology of cryptosporidiosis in humans and animals. Microbes and Infection,* **6**: 773-785.

Rodríguez Diego, J., Abreu, J. R., Pérez, E., Roque, E. and Cartas, O. 1991. Presence of *Cryptosporidium* in buffaloes (*Bubalus bubalis*) in Cuba. Rev. *Salud. Anim,* **13**: 78–80.

Santin, M., Trout, J. M., Xiao, L., Zhou, L., Greiner, E.and Fayer, R. 2004. Prevalence and age-related variation of *Cryptosporidium species* and genotypes in dairy calves.*Veterinary Parasitology,* **122**: 103-117.

Sherchand, J. B. and Shrestha, M. P.1996. Prevalence of *Cryptosporidium* infection and diarrhoea in Nepal.*J.Diarrhoeal Dis Res,* **14** (2): 81-84

Siwila, J. and Mwape, K. E. 2012. Prevalence of *Cryptosporidium spp.* and *Giardia duodenalis* in pigs in Lusaka, Zambia.*Onderstepoort Journal of Veterinary Research,* **79** (1).

Snelling, W. J., Xiao, L., Pierres, G., Lowery, C. J., Moore, J. E., Rao, J. R., Smyth, S., Millar, B. S., Rooney, P. J., Matsuda, M., Kenny, F., Xu, J.and. Dooley, J. S. G 2007. Cryptosporidiosis in developing countries. *J. Infect Developing countries,* **1** (3): 242-256.

Taherkhani, H., Fallah, M., Jadidian, K., and Vaziri, S., 2007. A study on the prevalence of *Cryptosporidium* in HIV positive patients. *J Res Health Sci,* **7** (2): 20-24

Vanopdenbosch, E., Wellemans, G., Dekegel, X., Strobbe, R., 1979. Neonatal calf diarrhoea: A complex etiology. *VI DiergTijdschr,* **48**: 512–526.

Venu, R., Latha, B. R., Basith, S. A., Raj, G. D., Sreekumar, C., and Raman, M., 2012. Molecular prevalence of *Cryptosporidium spp.* In dairy calves in southern states of India. *Veterinary Parasitology*, **188**: 19-24.

Woods, K. M., Nesterenko, M. V., Upton, S. J., 1996. Efficacy of 101 antimicrobials and other agents on the development of *Cryptosporidium parvum* in vitro. *Annal Tropical Medicine Parasitology*, **90**: 603–615.

Xiao, L., Fayer, R., Rayan, U., Upton, S. J. 2004. *Cryptosporidium* Taxonomy: recent advances and implications for public health. *Clinical Microbiol. Reviews*, **17** (1): 72-97.

Yatswako, S., Faleke, O. O., Gulumbe, M. L., and Daneji, A. I., 2007. *Cryptosporidium oocysts* and *Balantidium coli* cysts in pigs reared semi-intensively in Zuru, Nigeria. *Pakistan Journal of Biological Sciences*, **10** (19): 3435-3439.

Zajac, A. M., and Conboy, G. A., 2006. Veterinary Clinical Parasitology. Blackwell Publishing, USA.

Zhang W. J., Xu, L. H., Liu, Y. Y., Xiong, B. Q., Zhang, Q. L., Li, F. C., Song, Q. Q., Khan, M. K., Zhou, Y. Q., Zhao, Mu. J., 2012. Prevalence of coccidian infection in suckling piglets in china. *Veterianry parasitology*, **190**: 51-55.

Annexes

Annex 1. List of Photographs

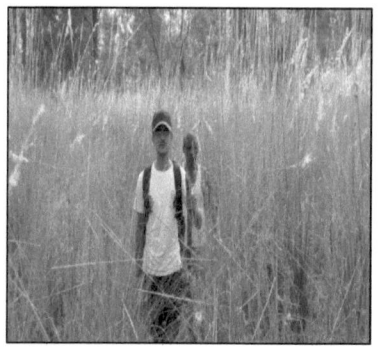

Searching for Wild buffalo

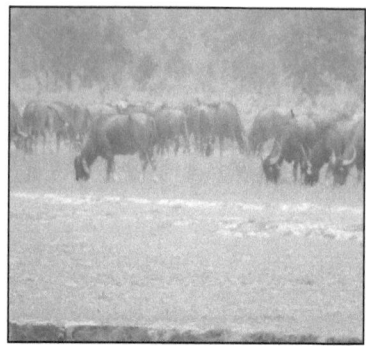

Herd of Wild water buffalo (Arna)

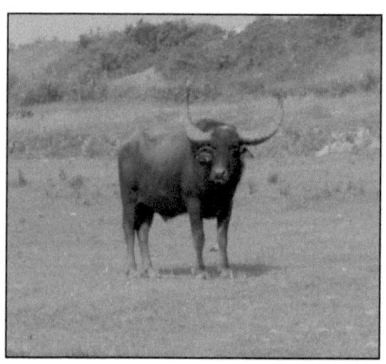

Solitary male

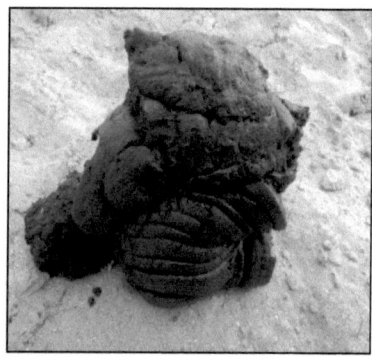

A single pile of fresh dung of wild water buffalo
(*Bubalus arnee*)

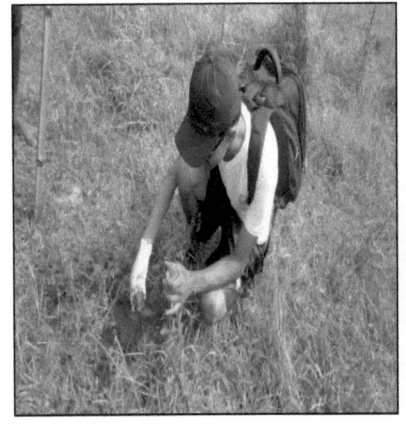

Sample Collection

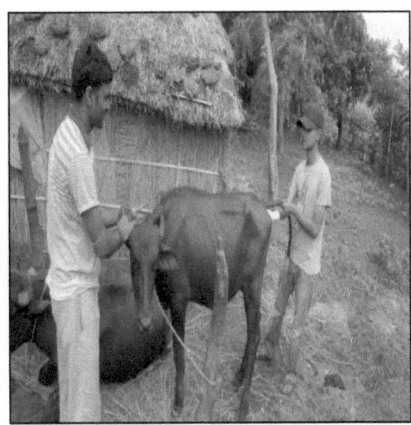

Per rectum collection of dung of domestic buffalo

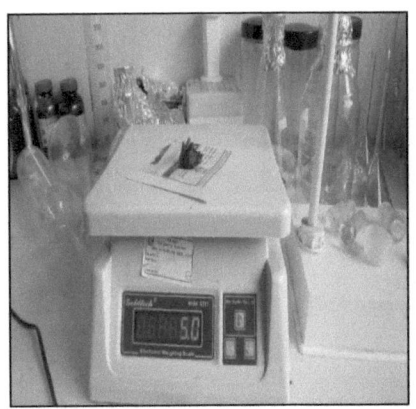

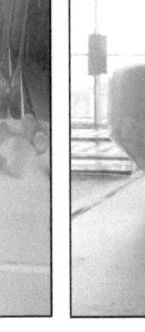

Weighing of Sample

Centrifugation of sample

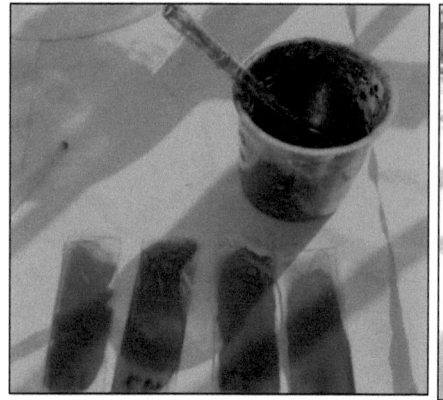
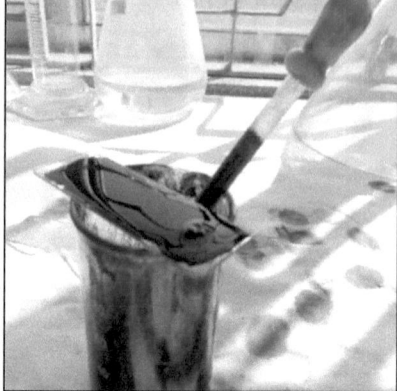

Carbolfuschin staining   Malachite green staining

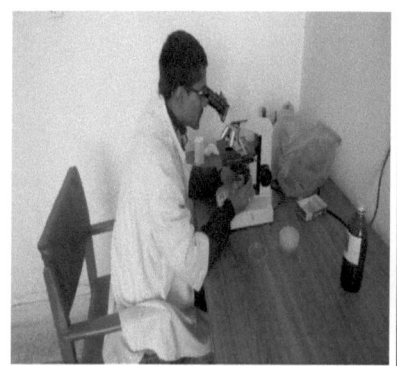
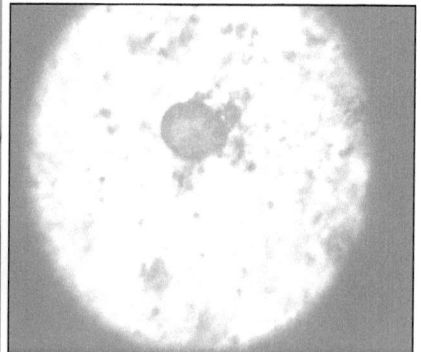

Microscopic examination   *Cryptosporidium spp*

Annex 2. Preparation of the reagents

1. CarbolFuchsin

To make 100 ml of CarbolFuchsin

Step 1:

Basic Fuchsin + Ethanol Solution A

(150 g) 1000 ml

Step 2:

Solution A + 5% Phenol Solution CarbolFuchsin

(10 ml) (90 ml)

2. 5% Malachite green, 5 g/l (0.5% w/v)

To make 1 liter of the solution, add 5 g of Malachite Green powder and make it upto 1 liter.

3. 1% Acid alcohol

Carefully add 20 ml hydrochloric acid to 1980 ml of absolute methanol and mix.

4. Supersaturated Salt solution

Add 393 gm of salt in 1 liter of distilled water intermittently, heat the solution and swirl during the procedure.